Alcoholism

Beating The Dreaded Drink

Written By
Alastair R Agutter

ALL RIGHTS RESERVE

PHOTOGRAPH COVER:

By Alastair R Agutter

www.alastairagutter.com

Copyright © Paperback Book First Edition 2014

PUBLISHED ON

First Published: 24th January 2014

BOOK PUBLISHERS

Create Space Independent Publishing - An Amazon Group Company

DISTRIBUTION

Paperback Book Edition for International Distribution

ISBN

ISBN-10: 149758437X

ISBN-13: 978-1497584372

ALL RIGHTS RESERVED

Introduction

Like many folk, I grew up surrounded by Alcohol, especially at Christmas time, and on special occasions.

Through the ages, alcohol has been a staple diet for many in cultures, and society. Wine especially, in Egyptian, Roman and Greek times, up to the current day.

In England, throughout the Centuries has there been much consumed, and as a result, of dysentery, in many larger communities such as Villages, Towns, and Cities. Where drink was consumed as ales, and malts, as part of their daily diet, as the water in those days, were too contaminated.

Today, I am pleased to see how society has evolved, where we can now enjoy water in its purist form, and where hygiene is very much a part of our everyday lives. But as we embrace many positives, as a result of human evolution, a more complex society, and standard of living has emerged.

Many describe alcoholism as a condition, or a disease, in our modern superficial society, where we can attach many tags, to events, or conditions, to satisfy ourselves, as to say, we understand. But that is not the case, it is so often a matter of seeking to ignore, or not venture further, into these habits, and events, that impact so many lives, and where, we fail to confront, or address them.

Today in Britain, the United States, and many other Countries in the World, We see disruption, and insular politics, where the real issues of the day, are not being addressed. In Britain we have a serious health problem regarding alcoholism, and yet politicians, and successive Governments, fail to serve the community, by bringing into check, some sensible and moral statutes of Law, in the interests of Health and Society. Government and Local Authorities in Britain know that alcoholism is a forever increasing problem. Politicians, and political parties, are reminded each day, by Medical Professionals and Enforcement agencies, namely the Police.

Yet politicians fail to act in the most honourable way, and legislate to curb today's society's ills, as a result of economic and corporate profitability demands before the health of a Nation!

This guide I hope will help folk identify their own issues, with alcohol consumption, and the reasons behind such events, where many are related to stress, in relationships, work environments, and financial pressures.

It deeply saddens me to see today, so many families, where Children are involved, breaking up, as a result of this social ill, engineered by a greed driven society, and negligent Governance.

I hope this short book and guide, will save many marriages, and relationships, and help find answers, and clarity, with an aim of serving the interests of the community. So folk, and families, can embark on a more loving, and successful path, in their lives and relationships.

It is very easy, for many to past judgement, or opinion, without fully understanding, and experiencing the problems. I often get animated, from hearing of Childcare experts, and related programmes on television regarding child behaviour, and care. Where none of the so called experts, have any idea about parenthood, and their views and suggestions, I find to be morally wrong, and offensive. Such irresponsible negligence should be held to account!

So I take you through this subject based on my personal experience of alcoholism the emotions and events regarding the dreaded drink. I am sharing with you, my life experiences, where I conquered alcoholism and to help explain in this short book, and guide. Where I have experienced first-hand such events in my life, that have resulted in the breaking down of relationships, heart ache, and so much more.

I admire folk, who are beginning to talk about conditions in their lives, one notably, Steve Fry, fighting depression, again a symptom described as an illness.

I dedicate this short book and guide, to every person, or family, that this short book and guide will help, to beat the dreaded drink. But also to my dearly loved wife (Christine), who endured many events in our marriage, where forgiveness is all I could every ask, even after 12 years of separation, where I miss her still every day, and where I only wish, I could turn the clock back.

Also to a man, who I met on my journey of life, called "Tony". Tony was a person I came to know who was suffering from mental illness, depression, and alcoholism. Who freed me from such a wasted cycle in my life, and where I never drank again. Thanks Tony!

Alastair R Agutter

Author

How The Hell Can You Help Someone, Who Will Not Help Themselves

One of my favourite films of all time was a Robert Redford Masterpiece, called "The River Runs Through it". It was a story of a small town in Montana, in the United States. Where, a River ran through the community, called "The Big Black Foot".

The true story back drop was around the 1930's if I recall, and there were two Sons of the local Presbyterian Church reverend. For film buffs, it was in fact, the first big film, where we really saw Brad Pitt, as a début. So for all Brad Pitt woman fans, it is a good excuse to watch the film, and to understand the story.

The two Brothers were taught fly-fishing by their Father, a noble pastime, and one of great skill, and where I often say to folk, when fly-fishing in the past, it is a time to rejuvenate ones soul!

As like all boys, they tasted life at an early age, and alcohol was just one part of it, like all of us do, if we are honest. Well, one of the Brothers went off to University, and the other, became a local newspaper journalist.

Well, in the film, there is a scene, where the two Brothers are fly-fishing with a guest. The day was hot, and their guest, had raided, and drank all the beer they were cooling by the water's edge. They found the guest, out like a light, as they say. Then as the two Brothers talked and reflected on their guest, the eldest Brother remarked, "How the hell can you help that son of a bitch". The younger Brother replied, "Perhaps it's the thought that someone is trying to help him".

Well, with alcoholism in a relationship, it is often a cry for help. For alcoholism is not a disease or some of form of rational definition, to departmentalize the problems, so society can draw some form of closure under the problem?

Excessive drinking is very often a form of self-medication, to escape pressures, and events, in a person's life, or relationship.

To reach such a point, it is where society, and people in relationships, needs to help each other, by talking and addressing the issues that result in drinking excessively.

So What Are The Causes of Drinking

Most excessive or heavy drinking is as a result of work circumstances, relationships, emotional stress, and the common denominator to all in most instances, is financial pressures.

In most cases, women tend to be more open, and can discuss matters with friends, and relatives. Where they can normally rationalize to coup, or deal with the situation, in a family relationship with others where women can work through the problem, such as alcoholism.

With our beloved women, this can very often be described as a reality check, and where there are very often friends, and family there in lives that can support them, and give encouragement in their hour of need.

Men are very often a different commodity, and here is the reason why? Most men are loyal and loving, however they can be foolish, and lose sight of the family unit at times, where judgement under such stress can be extremely clouded.

However in most cases for the love of a wife and Children, when men are confronted with financial these problems or work related pressures they tend not to discuss them, but try to find a way to work things out themselves.

Why do they not share, or discus the problems?

Normally, it is as a result of loving their wife, and children, so much, that they keep such problems secret, to avoid causing worry, and anxiety to the ones they love.

Intimate relationships failing between couples, can also spark desperation, where alcohol can become a companion, where they end up in the pub, or work late, or drink in the evenings at home, and fall asleep.

A sexual relationship in a marriage is important to most men, and if such a relationship becomes stale, they can reside themselves into a bout of depression, and only motivated by drinking, as a form of medication, to keep the drive going, to continue to work, and pay the bills.

When a relationship is under stress with financial worries, it is not a time to cast negative criticism to the partner, as this just further impacts the problem. Also in a relationship, where the husband has the problem with drinking, it is not something the woman should discuss with relatives, or friends. As there is always at least someone, or more, who have problems of their own, and capitalise on your misfortunes, to stoke the fire of the problem (jealousy) to make themselves feel better. It is a bitter and wicked act, but sadly in today's society it is not uncommon.

A marriage, or relationship, as a family, and especially with children, with these problems, needs to be resolved between yourselves, and not external parties.

Speaking from personal experience, my ex-mother in law did not particularly like me, and the opportunity to create a rift, or to encourage the breakdown of our relationship was encouraged, and at every opportunity. So if you want to keep your marriage, you have to work through it together, and support your loved one.

If you feel in truth, you cannot stick together, and work through these difficult times, you then have to look at your marriage, and ask yourself truthfully, at the first hurdle, or crisis, what drew you both together, in the first place.

When such events happen, where a partner is suffering, and drinking excessively, the best thing to do, is to sit down together, cuddle and talk. The holding of a hand, and listening to a stressed loved one, is a sign of support, and encouragement, and such a kindness, is forever remembered, especially if the partner with the problem is the male.

All men are strong, and most with a good heart, the expression of emotions is not a weakness, more of the case that your relationship has become extremely close, and if this is the case, you need to know regardless of all his friends, or yours. If you love each other, you should be each other's best friends.

By talking, and supporting each other, you can both rationally look at things both together, and work through the problems. Where you can evaluate the financial pressures, and begin to look at what is exactly necessary, and other commitments that are more luxuries, and not necessities.

You will be amazed, by giving this love, and support, how much pressure is released, and taken off of the suffering partner. Your partner does not need medical help, this is important to know. For any Doctor worth his, or her sort, will tell your partner suffering, that the consumption of excessive alcohol, is a form of self-medication, where your partner, for those brief few hours of intoxication, are trying to take away, and escape from the misery, and heartache in his, or her life.

Be completely supportive, and work together. Find extra time for each other, and spend more intimate moments together, and begin to enjoy yourselves again. For as like any addition be it drinking or smoking. The best way of giving up, and the healthiest way and where there any cravings, is by replacing them, with intimate sexual moments.

There is no bigger turn off, than seeing your loved one drunk, unless your relationship is very strong. On the odd occasions, my wife was drunk, from a girl's nights out, and she was completely legless and virtually carried in by her girlie friends, it was more of a question of concern for her, as I loved every part of her.

If you have a relationship where you literally worship the ground a person walks on as I did with my wife. Then you can get through it. We did in our relationship several times, for I was always under tremendous pressure, developing new products, and services.

Our relationship ended in the end, not from my wife giving up on me, but I became so depressed, as work dried up from the Dot.Com crash, and started drinking heavily again. I loved her so much, and the Children, I just had to leave, and walk away, as I did not want the insults, or the arguments, or worst still the fights.

Alcohol is a really ugly, nasty poison, and in truth, I hate it today, and even the thought of it makes me feel sick. However, as a social animal, I have no hang ups with others drinking, or going out socializing. In fact I enjoy life so much more, as I retain all my brain cells that I need, and wake up without a hangover, or feeling extremely ill.

The Symptoms of Heavy Drinking And The Risks

When heavy drinking starts, it truly is the road to ruin, and can jeopardise not only your family, but your career, and friends.

When you start to crave a drink every day, to get by, and any opportunity to have a drink, that is when you have a problem, and it needs to be addressed immediately.

With the support of your loved one, and discussing problems, and pressures, have you a chance.

If you also find yourself buying drink, to have at home, and then stopping off at the pub, and worst still driving home, you are not only endangering the future of your family, your career, but others lives, by getting into a lethal weapon, for that is exactly what a car is and you could face a driving ban, and worse still a custodial sentence!

If you are desperate for a drink, literally pinch yourself, and stop, for it could end up in arguments, and fights with your loved ones, and as a result of again, irresponsible policies in Britain, by negligent politicians, the landscape today, will result in arrest, court, separation and more broken lives and where your children are affected!

Cure and Conquering The Addiction

As I say, there is no point going to a Doctors, they cannot help. Only to point out, as mentioned before, you are drinking, as self-medication. More pills, and medication, is not the answer either, you cannot beat depression, as it is not an illness, but a frame of mind, due to relationships and circumstances.

The secret to discouraging drink is to set a target each day, and avoid drinking full stop! Literally say to yourself, it is killing you, and your relationship. When you have another hangover, it is seriously the time, to look in the mirror.

Then get the first coffee, or tea down you, or even orange juice, and think yeap, I have a family I love, a wife that is supporting, and talking to me over the pressures and problems, and we are doing something about the financial pressures together, as a supportive family.

Make time for the family, realise what you have, and get out, rather than sit in front of a television. Get the kids out with you, on walks, and do things as a family. A day out with a family, is cheaper than a week's drinking, and believe it or not, you will be financially far better off, and having fun with your loved ones.

Another way to conquer the dreaded drink is to do what I done and this was by sheer co-incidence and it was the changing moment in my life, and see it through!

I was asked by a friend, who I had befriended, who was suffering badly from alcohol and depression, and for some reason that day in my life. I just did not feel like a drink, myself. I had just been to newsagents, and bought a new computer magazine that morning, and my friend with me, asked to go to the local pub, that was a decent place. But instead of a drink, I just felt like an orange juice and lemonade, as I sat in a warm friendly atmosphere, and read my magazine, while keeping Tony Company.

After his first pint, he was still civil and jovial. The second pint, he appeared relaxed. On the way back to where he lived, to make sure he was OK, he wanted to stop off at another pub, and I agreed. I remember again, I just wanted a coke, and he began his third pint, and then I saw the demon drink appear. He became loud, his expression and eyes changed, and he became belligerent, and boisterous. For the first time in my life, I was looking at me, and immediately thought of the many years, I had put my dear loving wife through. It made me feel sick and in truth, I did not like myself one bit.

The day I walked out for the love of my family and when I wanted to return, my wife in a conversation said no! At that time of stress and anxiety, I took that as red, and respected her decision. My deepest regret to this day, is that we never talked, or worked through the problem together, on that occasion, as I have suggested. As a stupid man some weeks later after the separation I received a note, with pictures of my family, and wife. I did not realise, it was a subtle signal to remind me, what I had given, up and lost but still there for me. But the words, never to come back, stuck in my stupid mind, and I did not understand these subtle gestures, of how our greatest equal, and best friends, often behave, our woman!

I have been in morning now for over 12 years, for the loss of my best friend, and soul mate. I would not want you, to reach that point, or make the same mistake in your relationship. Every day, I think of my wife, and every day, I serve that sentence of loss!

If you have a close and trusted friend and have the courage to go out with them but do not drink yourself you will see the changes in them from a heavy drinking session and you will then see the demon first hand, that you are putting your loved ones through.

Spending that critical time with my friend Tony and seeing him change that evening was a changing moment in my life For I sat in silence, and looked out into the dark of the night that evening, and realised from the demon drink, what a disgusting poison, it is and how it destroys lives.

The following day, Tony called for me, and wanted to have a New Year's Day drink. I agreed to walk up the road with him, to ensure he was all right, but when he asked me into his local pub, I declined, and that day, was the last day, I saw Tony, and for his friendship, as sad as it was, he helped me, and for that I will be forever in his debt.

People say leopards never change their spots; well people can change, and evolve. I have not drunk since that day the 1st of January 2006. Some would say many could be lured back to drinking from pressure, but in truth, the pressure in the last 5 years, running a large business, with many staff dependent, on myself, and fighting lawyers, suppliers, and landlords, working 24/7 and where I collapsed with exhaustion. At no time, was I ever tempted.

My best friend still today, in the form of a drink, is a cup of tea. Or, when I am out socialising, an orange juice and lemonade just suits me fine. Knowing, I am retaining every grey cell I have, enjoying the company on those evenings, and waking the next day, without a hangover and not feeling like crap!

Help and Advice

There are always plenty in this World to pass opinion and criticism, but many have not experienced the pressures one is enduring, or have the common decency to stop and put their brains in gear.

The only person that can beat the dreaded drink and with love and support from loved ones is you. There is no one else!

Perhaps, looking at the state of our Western Society today, perhaps a sobering act and tonic to kick the habit would be to go out to any large city or town sober, on a Saturday night late. Where you will witness and see first-hand human behaviour of the worst kind from drug addition of drink and even embarrassing to watch.

Sadly there are many in our society, that are driven solely by money and brewers are very ruthless in marketing, to the point of where alcoholism is an accepted part of Western Society.

But the damage it is causing is mind blowing and where most twenty year olds today, will either die, or be in need of transplants before they reach 40 years I age, from heart disease, or liver failure.

Alcohol is a poison and it kills thousands of brain cells and can cause irreparable damage to your heart. Even after giving up excessive drinking, history of alcohol abuse can be found even decades later from medical examination and tests.

Sadly in our western society, we do not see responsible governance, to clamp down on irresponsible vendors, who encourage and offer many incentives to buy and consume more alcohol. Supermarkets in respect of this serious social ill are certainly not friends to any of us in society.

Governments take no action, as they are keener on collecting taxes from the supermarkets or fines through the courts and that is the reality.

In these tough and uncertain times, there is even greater reason to give up drinking, as no job, or career is certain anymore, and every penny is needed to secure the well-being of your family and loved ones.

As a parent with Children, there is nothing more embarrassing to your Children, than to see a parent drunk. The other consideration and reality is you are introducing your children to this social ill that they will eventually adopt.

Drinking is just a frame of mind, nobody needs it to have a good time and by avoiding it, your Children will grow up respecting you and your loved one, with fond memories, rather than haunting ones caused from drinking.

For me, my life has changed completely, and I hope this

guide helps you. I have a young Daughter who is my World, and now my best friend, where we spend quality time together, and she is never fearful, or intimated, or nervous, as she has a Daddy that loves, cares and makes her laugh.

My close friends know the real me, and always talk at important times in their lives, some are Girlfriends in the truest sense as friends, having their own families, and where we discuss Children, and daily lives, and support each other. And for my dear wife who I still love to this day. I always remember the words she once said that haunt me, "you are a lovely man, if only you wouldn't drink, and a wonderful Father".

Drinking in any form when you have to put a glass to your lips is a losers game, that first drink might not be the one, but it is the start to an eventual road to ruin. Drink will eventually kill you in some way, if you do not kick the habit.

When I see people today drinking, I truthfully think how sad!

Serving The Community

I am always available for Motivational Speeches, to help community members as they confront the serious problems of alcohol in society. Police, Local Governments, Charities and Commercial Organizations, I can avail my time to help address and deal with this social ill that is affecting too many lives in the work place, personal performance, and family relationships.

Especially the Police, as these brave men and woman face terrible stressful events every day of their lives, and if I can provide positive help, comfort and support, to ensure they are in the right place, and frame of mind. They will then be able to help themselves, as well as serve the community positively, and safely.

This publication is available 'FREE' on request to Police, Local Government, National Governments, Charities, and Organizations in PDF form. To help Communities, and people fight this dreadful social ill, affecting so many lives in our society.

I can be contacted by the following means:-

Web site: www.alastairagutter.com

Email: info@alastairagutter.com

About The Author

Alastair R Agutter was born in Farnborough, England in 1958 to English parents.

He is a freelance (self-employed) Writer, Philosopher, Logistician, Theoretical Physicist, Author, Publisher, Naturalist, Environmentalist, Computer Scientist, Creative Digital Artist and Proud Father of Five Children.

His first printed book was "The Discus Fish" in 1988, covering the successful breeding and rearing in captivity the beautiful Symphysodon. A native species found in the Great River Amazon and adjoining tributaries and Rivers in South America. The publication has since been re-written and updated in 2013 for Kindle and other tablet devices, as a Digital Publication.

He is a passionate advocate for the environment and a naturalist at heart, with a great respect for all living creatures and with founding principles for the preservation of all species, many sadly under threat today from climate change. He believes there is no reason why the human race cannot learn from quantum mechanics, and co-exist with the environment and all living species on Earth.

To find out more, about the author's, new up and coming book releases, and to get the latest news please visit www.alastairagutter.com

AUTHOR'S OTHER BOOKS

Available online and through reputable High Street Book Store Retailers World-Wide

I become inspired to write books, when I encounter a subject that I am passionate about and where I believe I can make some positive humble contribution to society.

The Discus Book – Hard Back

The Discus Book – Kindle Digital Edition

The Discus Book – Paper Back

Children's Weebies Early Reading English - Kindle Digital

Children's Weebies Early Reading English – Paper Back

The News 2013 Almanac - Kindle Digital Edition

The News 2013 Almanac - Paper Back Book

My England A Broken Nation - Kindle Digital Edition

My England A Broken Nation – Paper Back Book

Beating The Dreaded Drink - Kindle Digital Edition

Beating The Dreaded Drink – Paper Back Book

Getting Inside Google's Head - Kindle Digital Edition

Getting Inside Google's Head – Paper Back Book

A Book For Celebrating Web Art – Kindle Digital Edition

A Book For Celebrating Web Art – Paperback

The Discus Book Special Edition – Kindle Digital Edition

The Discus Book Special Edition - Paperback

The Discus Book 2nd Edition – Kindle Digital Edition

The Discus Book 2nd Edition - Paperback

All of the Author's books are available online through reputable books sellers, such as the Author's publishers and distributors Amazon.Com, or other long established booksellers online such as Barnes & Noble, for Nook Digital Editions.

The books are also available in Paper Back through reputable Retail High Street book stores internationally.

www.alastairagutter.com

Official Web Site of the

Author

BEATING THE DREADED DRINK BOOK

By Alastair R Agutter

www.alastairagutter.com

Copyright © Paperback Book First Edition 2014

PUBLISHED ON

First Published: 24th January 2014

BOOK PUBLISHERS

Create Space Independent Publishing - An Amazon Group Company

DISTRIBUTION

Paperback Book Edition for International Distribution

ISBN

ISBN-10: 149758437X

ISBN-13: 978-1497584372

ALL RIGHTS RESERVED

Printed in Great Britain
by Amazon